LOVE IN A TIME OF LAMENT

For Jeff with admiration for the
Bayliss family —
Blessings, Regina

ALSO BY RENNIE McQUILKIN

An Astonishment and an Hissing
North Northeast
We All Fall Down
Counting to Christmas
Learning the Angels
Passage
Getting Religion
Private Collection
First & Last
The Weathering: New & Selected Poems
Visitations
Going On
A Quorum of Saints
Dogs
North of Eden: New & Collected Poems
Afterword
The Readiness
Seabury Seasons
Coming Through
The Rounding
The Holding

LOVE IN A TIME OF LAMENT

An Alzheimer's Memoir

Poems by

Rennie McQuilkin

Rennie McQuilkin (signature)

Antrim House
Bloomfield, Connecticut

ISBN: 979-8-9865522-7-9

Library of Congress Control Number: 2023932645

First Edition, 2023

Printed & bound by Ingram Content Group

Book design by Rennie McQuilkin

Front cover enamel by Yvonne Gaudriot

Back cover photograph by Eleanor McQuilkin Burns

Back cover painting ("Nobska Lighthouse") by Sarah McQuilkin

Antrim House
860.519-1804
AntrimHouseBooks@gmail.com
www.AntrimHouseBooks.com
400 Seabury Dr., #5196, Bloomfield, CT 06002

For Sarah, forever

PREFACE

In addition to new work, the considerably revised poems in this collection have been selected from two of my previous books, *The Rounding* and *The Holding*. They focus on my belovèd Sarah's battle with Alzheimer's, both before and after her move to Seabury's memory support center and now, tragically, refer to her passage into another world. I offer these poems as a tribute to my gentle and great-hearted partner of sixty-two years. My heart is broken, and I am consoled only by knowing it was her wish to "go home" and by the serenity with which she departed. In the hearts of all those who knew her, she rests in peace and joyful memory.

Rennie McQuilkin
Bloomfield, CT
April, 2023

TABLE OF CONTENTS

I. ALZHEIMER'S

II. HOME

III. AFTERWORLD

Though we need to weep your loss,
You dwell in that safe place in our hearts,
Where no storm or night or pain can reach you.

John O'Donohue

LOVE IN A TIME OF LAMENT

I. ALZHEIMER'S

The Terror

At three a.m. she wakes me, crying out
in a voice so deep and stricken I barely know it:
"We're losing someone, losing!" As if drowning,

she gasps for air, clutching
so hard I might be a spar floating mid-ocean.
Telling her she has had a bad dream will not do,

nor my embraces. She holds harder, cries
"Don't leave me, don't go!" I say no, I will stay,
try to help if she will say who we are losing.
"Don't you know? How could you not?"

She stares at something fearful.
At length she begins to breathe more slowly, deeply,
and falls asleep, her mild breathing like the lapping
of ocean waters quelled on a quiet shore . . .

In the morning she has no memory
of her night terror. We drink coffee, chat amicably.
I read aloud to her, as always. But I am undone.
All day I have been redoubling gifts of love for her.

Her Family

She startles me from sleep by appearing
in the wee hours dressed for travel,
announcing she has just seen a child home.

I hold her a long time, lost but knowing
she is becoming the essence of herself:
love beyond boundaries.

Next morning she sleeps late, curled warmly.
At breakfast, she engages in a playful
naming of birds at the feeder:

Popeye for the gilt male goldfinch,
Olive for the protective, more secret female.
She is crossing over. All things are family.

Loss

There was a time when loss was
merely a sad case.
But these days Loss is capitalized.

Just now it's your spectacles –
brand new trifocals allowing you
to stay in touch – that are lost
"forever" you say through sobs.
How much of you keeps vanishing!

When we find the glasses teetering
on the top edge of a window sash
next to the Peace Lily you keep
from wilting away, you sob again
with delight.

You and I vow to be vigilant.
Whatever losses accumulate,
we will cling to our cliff,
keep our fingernails in fighting trim.

The Waiting

First thing in the morning she's tightly swaddled
in blankets pulled around her,
seems bound for the Egyptian Underworld . . .

Happily, the wraps are closer to a silk moth's
cocoon. The slightest stir's within.
I rise and wait, relying on coffee and biscuit,

collecting the least crumbs
with a fingertip, tasting them, savoring
all that is left – most of all her, remembering

how she reached deep in the womb of a ewe,
turned the lamb, pulled him out by the forelegs;
how she dug buried spuds, held them up to view.

I am willing her to break free of her wrappings,
brighten, returned to me to taste the elixir I offer
and drink day in once more.

Joy

In the midwinter desperation
of a ride to Emergency, distressed
at every jounce, she cries out in joy,
staring wide-eyed
at the day's blue emptiness of sky –

"Oh look, how white the moon!"
She holds up a figment of it
between her thumb and forefinger
and blows on it like sending the fluff
of a dandelion sailing into heaven.

February 1

Praised be the curl of blizzard-bent snow
on the roof across the pond –
signature of the immense Beyond;

also the optimistic Groundhog dug in,
warmed by the big snow, dreaming of Spring,
no interest in tomorrow's shadow;

also the way you and I, my love – *rabbit rabbit* –
emerge from opposite ends of our digs,
emerge at just the same time, without a shadow

of discord. May this predict a fruitful warmth,
a fiercely temperate time equal to the storm.
Call it Love.

Be Mine

After days of rain, the roof across the way
is putting on airs. The dark dampness
at edges of each bright shingle could be
the lead dividing antique window glass.

Too fancy. I prefer the sharp triangles,
squares and circles of sun-cast shadow
on clapboard, various as the cutouts
of the happy child you were all yesterday,

preparing valentines. I learn from you,
my love, say nothing fancy, just "Be mine"
as you emerge from your remove.

A Valentine for Sarah

We had a falling out last night.
This morning I try to right myself
but as with all my falls it's hard
to haul up, put a best foot forward.

I take courage from the weather
that has taken a turn for the warmer.
In Pete's Pond, breeze-blown ripples
of melt must be riding over sinking ice.

Hopeful Painteds under the weather
all winter in muck like my own
are no doubt climbing to deadwood
to drink in sun, stick their necks out,
long red-and-yellow-striped necks,
taking a chance one more time.

I too. A falling out requires a falling
in. Forgive, forgive.

Distribution

The forecast calls for a front
but today's sky is cloudless
and she as well
after yesterday's storm.

I am reminded of my first car –
how rain made the distributor
misfire, the cylinders sputtering
until a drying sun perfected them.

Today she distributes blessings.
She knows me. No curses.
She praises my efforts and all
the nosegay colors of the garden.

How I want this not to end,
no storm, nothing
but this perfect moment.

The Touching

*She's touched your perfect body with
her mind.*

> "Suzanne," Leonard Cohen

After being savaged by surgery
I didn't want anyone seeing my
body's ruin, not even you, my dear.

But you thought otherwise, wiser
despite your forgetfulness. Deeper
than logic, you wanted us as before.

You said you'd only take a shower
if we went under the water together.
There, both of us naked as newborns,

you touched my imperfect body with
your impaired mind and loving hands,
touched me all over, making me shine.

Traveler

She sees her reflection in
the sheen of my cellphone,
toys with her bobbed hairdo,
as if in a car mirror,

nearing a special destination.
Hers now is a home beyond
this place she is dying to leave.

She smiles, purses lips, applies
imaginary Revlon.
I'm with her on this final ride.

Anniversary Song

We watch two doves on a rooftop
standing chest to chest, tall necks
braiding, touching beak to beak,
cooing in the aftermath of love,

recalling us, years ago
after the dance of our bodies –
ourselves again, seeing eye to eye.

Now he flies off in excited circles
while she does the Lambeth Walk
down the ridge of the roof,
barely glancing at him but aware
somewhere deep within that it will

soon be time to prepare, arranging
what he will bring – twine and twigs,
bits of moss, fur, and torn clothing –
piling them around herself,
making a nest shaped like a dove.

We too, my love,
were part of the great adventure
and celebrate it today.

Clair de Lune

Your hands shake, seeming to seek
what's lost . . . But no, this is not the palsy
that accompanies dementia, undoing me,
but in tune with Debussy
who fills the room, moving from your hands
to your whole conducting self. Your lips
tremble an iteration of the harmony;
your feet two-step.
How a darkened mind is enlightened by music!

Learning

"I hate you!" she says,
like a child loving a parent
so fiercely
she spats if the parent
demands.
        I am learning
to hear beneath her words,
let her rest, begin again
in love.

Sentence

She asks if I could . . .
would I see if . . .
and looks blankly beyond,
can't end a sentence.
I nod. I hold her hand.

Good Morning

Midmorning she stays wrapped in blankets.
"I'm scared," she says. I stroke her hair.
We talk about what frightens her.
She doesn't know where she is or how she got here.
We reconstruct and she stirs, though unconvinced.

She emerges from her tight wrapping,
widens her eyes, looks at what she tries to know.
When I say who I am, she shakes her head,
but blinks, perhaps hoping to renew
our acquaintance.

"Good morning, my love."
"Good morning," she whispers uncertainly
and moves closer, lifts her pajama sleeves
like brilliant wings.

Time Change

I've "fallen back," floating
in an otherworldly hour of
loaned time.
Now a door-creak, and I see

a slice of light . . .
Slowly she comes into focus –
a wide set of eyes, a broad smile,
a sort of 17th Century angel
peering around a bank of cloud,

one of God's choristers come to
welcome me to Heaven. Instead,
her lovely earthly voice wishes me
"Happy Sunday." I've come through
another night. Praise the Lord.

Zebra

You want and want to "go home,
get out of this place!" I reason,
say it's time for bed,
but you insist, voice rising to crisis:
"Home, home, home! I want to go
to the car." I say it makes no sense –
this is our home. But you insist.
And I agree to take a night drive home

to "the zoo." Out of the underground
garage we go, turn onto Prospect . . .
"There they are," you chant –
ornamental cows in the unlikely pasture
of someone's yard, brighter than night
in their DayGlo colors, horned, uddered,
all but mooing. You moo back.

And at the far end of the herd
the strange one you love does more
than moo in his zoot suit of black & white
stripes with a lei of plastic sunflowers.
The zebra neighs like a trombone,
I know from the way you respond.
You open your arms to take him to you.
"Home, home," you sing happily, returning
with the stuffed animal you have in mind.

Underworld

The day it was final – you'd have to go
to The Meadows for memory support,
I gave blood, and on my way home,
I lost my wallet, that proof I existed.

I can bear the loss of my outer self
like Osiris, whose dismembered parts
were slowly collected and puzzled together.
Little by little, my credit cards, license, etc.
have been replaced, all but the photos,

which kept you with me, my love – you
at three, pigtailed, wide-smiling; you waving
from South Beach; you remaking the world
at your easel . . .
so much of you gone with my wallet –

and you yourself no longer with me.
Like Osiris, whose most vital part could not
be found, though outwardly he seemed intact,
I must spend my days in the underworld,
from which I'll be given only temporary release.

To Sarah in Memory Care

Back then I was at Fort Leonard Wood
(Fort Lost in the Woods)
in the Badlands of southern Missouri.

I was without you, lost, living only for
mail call, your words lifted hand to hand
to me in the back row of the barracks,

raw recruit. How I relished your letters,
feasting on the future. On my first leave
I'd fly to you back east. "Hoping you

haven't forgotten. . ." I wrote, and trekked
half a mile through Badlands weather
to the nearest mailbox.

Here we are again, you in Memory Care
and I lost, remembering and remembering.
When I can come, I hope you'll know me.

Sing-along

Limping, cane in hand, to Memory Care
after too hot a day for November, cold now,
I try to avoid stepping on a host of worms,
their pink skin turned white and shriveled.

Canaries in a mine. I enter one
dedicated to finding brillance buried in
the ore of dementia. I wear hope
like a headlamp, looking for signs of clarity

in the dark confines of my dear one's mind,
her head downcast at today's sing-along.
Please, love, give me a sign you remember.
Oh sing, sing a song from the gone days,

a bright seam of music to tell me not all is lost –
those walls of darkened mind will not fall in.

On the Use of Song

When I was nine, seventeen-year locusts
left empty husks on a backyard sycamore,

a memory too close to the newest truth –
the blank look on my belovèd's face.

And yet I hear her bright voice now,
pure among elders singing in The Meadows.

Locusts, free of their husks, electrify the last
of the year. My belovèd too has risen from

her broken case,
refuses not to be, insists on song.

Natural History

When I visited yesterday,
her feet were bare where she lay
abed, eyes closed, barely covered.
This was too much like a gurney.

I forced socks and slippers on her
and urged. She gripped her walker
unhappily, pushed off, half asleep,
to visit the goldfish I recommended.

Watching them fantail, suddenly
she laughed and fannywagged back.
On to the parakeets squawking.
She answered them raucously

and asked for *Wind in the Willows*.
I read the part when Mole comes out
from his underground home,
meets the Water Rat,

and goes boating down the first river
he has ever seen, taking a turn sculling.
She leaned forward, rowed and rowed,
was twelve again, back on Silver Lake.

The Coughing

Sadly alone, I think how much
you'd enjoy this with me –
sitting pretty in the catbird seat
of the sun room, watching a jay
eye to eye, close to the morning
sun and meadows, tassels of what's-it
(you'd know) frosted in honor of fall,
and All Hallows just ahead.
The jay is playful, biting a gilt leaf
and tossing it like salt over its shoulder.
Joyful on this cold day,
I'd best toss salt myself, in light of
your fearful coughing in Memory Care.
You'll be fine, if our paper birch is any
indication – they haven't come yet
to cut it down. It still holds up the Vs
of its catkins. Just so, may you go on
and on: may your coughing be like that
of the cold car I hear, just about to start.

The Visit

Armistice Day, 2022

You saved it, convinced the town
to let the old cast iron bridge stand
over the Farmington, not go the way
of Iron Horse Boulevard which it abuts –

no "iron horses" run there these days.
Not a trace of railway track is left,
and no depot, just a yuppie burger joint.

You saved that bridge
from also going under. It stands, vestige
of a past we wish for more than ever.

Now the Memory Care bus takes you
and other wheelchaired patients to what
has become the Bridge of Flowers,
except it's November – no flowers line it
when you line up for a group photo.

No flowers, no bird song
except for your wide and blossoming smile
and the old-time tune you let loose.
Far off we hear the hooting of an iron horse.

Forest Bathing

for Nurse Ashley and Sarah

You hate showers, must be dragged into the stall.
This morning I find you huddled in a dark corner
rather than be stripped and forced under a torrent
of water. You say you just want to "get out"
and ask if I could take you for a walk.
Easier said, since the door to the enclosed garden
is alarmed. But one of the nurses understands
the fierce need that today makes you bridle
when I say it's time to do morning exercises.
You have no interest in exercises. You want out.

Nurse Ashley finds you a coat and silences
the alarm. We walk in a circle like caterpillars
around the rim of a bowl until you say, "Oh look,"
stopping by ground cover, some low-growing kind
of juniper, I think. The tips of its green needles
are tinted blue like the tall Christmas tree within,
one of the things you love most in your new place.

Suddenly your knuckled face relaxes, lets me in
the way the garden's December trees with spring buds
are letting you in. And I understand
why the Japanese consider "forest bathing" to be a way
for the spirit to restore itself.

"Now we can go back in," you say,
and we do and you exercise exuberantly.

Noëling, 105th St., 1960

Thanks to James Rhodes for an assist

Do you remember, my love, how
across an alley fouled by garbage,
behind a cracked window
with one plywood pane, reggae
blasted on that Christmas Eve?

And how a hand strung lights on a
spindly tree? Blinking blue & red
lights bobbed everywhichway.
Then the hand produced a tin star,

which rose, paused a moment,
and proceeded
as if looking for the perfect spot –
stopped, and hovered high up.

Do you remember how right after,
we went out to West End Ave.
and gave ten to a Salvation Army
bell-ringer, kept just enough to buy
a lopsided pine of our own?

Home, we laid a boy doll under it
on a bed of excelsior and alongside,
a toy panda in place of a lamb,
and knelt down to string popcorn.

Christmas Tree

Today, with first snow decorating fields
of dark shingle on the roof of Memory Care,
is the day to buy you a foot-high Xmas tree

sprinkled with small white lights, plant it
on your bureau, high place you might see
as Tyrolean, full of the sound of music.

How you redo things in your distraction
is a blessing. I'd crawl into your mind, share
a world more bright than the one I'm in.

The Gift, Christmas Morning

On this frozen monastic morning without you
after days of terrifying winds tearing into us,
I want you
to hear the gracious bubbling of the porridge
I would serve you were you here. I want you

to see the bulging-open, Christmas-red amaryllis
and puffed-up pigeons, fat to fend off the cold
on a roof across the pond. Their soft burbling is
in tune with the bubbling of water bearing life to
winter-stilled koi under a sheltering shed of ice.

The lively waterflow creates a clearing, at its edge
a scintillant serration of ice glittering like a star.
I want you here to share this morning,
this Christmas gift. Here, my love, I give it to you.

Stay

The figure a poem makes [is] . . .
a momentary stay against confusion.

Robert Frost

To create a momentary stay against
confusion in the mind of my dear wife
by which I am undone,
I read *Wind in the Willows* to her,
not the 1001 stories Scheherazade tells
to prevent her demise – still, tale on tale

of the Water Rat, that would-be poet,
and the Mole, his underground friend
who has come up from his burrow
and though his mind is not as sharp as
his earth-pushing nose, is wholly charming.

They lose their way in the Wild Wood,
but are saved from a wintry fate
by the powerful Badger, who warms them,
feeds them, and tucks them in for the night.

My dear one and I are, of course,
the characters, saved from loss for now
by joy of the story.

II. HOME

January 22, 2023

My Dearest Sarah,

I am trying to enjoy this new day, my love. I slept through a good part of the night, up just twice, and am drinking new Verona coffee, strong. The amazingly tall amaryllis is at long last budding like a loosening fist—unlike my fist, which is clubbed against Situation – ours, my dearest. Since you contracted Covid, there is so much I don't know. Is Mozart playing on your Sirius, or your beloved Debussy? And your amaryllis, that twin of mine, is it too coming into its own? Have the nurses watered it? And you – have you been eating enough to keep yourself going? I hope you got the stuffed zebra I sent over for you to have and hold in place of me, and the picture of our Robin with that hen roosting on his head the way you roost in mine. How I love writing these letters to you as I used to when I was in the army and you at Skidmore! But running my hands over the keyboard is not like holding you to me. When I can finally visit, we will make up for lost time.

Your adoring husband,
Rennie

P.S. Today's ditty:

May you enjoy this snow
before tomorrow's sleet,
your blue eyes widening,
watching flakes, first time
ever. Such beauty so new.

The Dispersing

St. Francis would love it. She gives away everything –
clothes I bring to replace what she disperses;
favorite bedtime animals and tiny blinking Xmas tree;
the food and juice she offers like alms for anyone who
will eat and drink what she will not. Pursing her lips,
she blows kisses to us, who know less than she
how little she needs, and how much.

What We Want

Preparing for our approaching demise
undoes me, the legalities of it, so many
calls to automatons, chats with invisible
'helpers" leaving me helpless.
Most of all I am undone by anguish
as I think of you, my love.
I am not Atlas enough to bear it –

how you also stagger under ministrations
at your new place: prodding needles,
this therapy, that therapy, meals and pills
forced on you when all you want, I too,
is for us to lie quietly together, a stroking,
looking out to the sky like our amarylli
opening and opening.

Two Statues

On my way to pulling on socks or making
poems or morning coffee, dear Sarah,
I pass the two small statues atop my bureau
and between them
my many hats compiled like nesting boxes.

I pay scant attention to the statues that wait
patiently to have their say – that softwood
Buddha from the many Buddhas given out
when our friend died, perhaps hoping
to show us the way;

and our black soapstone copy of Barlach's
"Doubting Thomas," a straight-backed Christ
lifting a bent-backed Thomas, who looks up
beseechingly to the Rabbi, anxious to believe.
I stop by him today, en route to quotidian things,

and feel my desire
to believe the Creed you have always repeated
while I've stood silent. Meanwhile the Buddha
is silent too. He seems to accept whatever is.
I would if I could, but I have no Negative Capability.

Which must be why I avoid the Barlach standing
higher than I. But like those hats compiled
next to the straight-backed Jesus, I'm always by Him,
doubting. My dear, I love how your faith sustains you
and will help you in the end. Please help me believe!

The Circling

Nineteen years ago, in her last days
at Christmas time, I gave my mother
a dozen large figures from Tanzania –

three magi, two shepherds, a villager,
the Holy Family, and three lambs,
some kneeling, others with bent knees
about to kneel, their black teak heads
seamless on brown acacia bodies.

I set them in a row on a narrow ledge
beside my mother's hospital bed
like a procession of penitents
or refugees, but no snipers, no strafing.

That was then. Dying was not endemic,
mongers of hate half asleep in their dens,
flowered Ukrainians festive at weddings,
and my wife still herself.

Today the figures came to light, lost
where Sarah stashed them before memory
faded. I place them in a Stonehenge circle,
the largest casting protective shadows over
the Child at the center, face licked by a lamb.

In my distraction, I see Sarah in the manger,
her future, like the Christ Child's, more dire
than I can bear. And more imminent.

Home

She tightens lips against crushed meds, spoonfuls of food,
straws pushed at her to offer lemonade . . . She is finding
her way home.

The Call

comes today, the one I have been dreading,
the words a blur: *crisis . . . dehydration . . .
severe . . . ambulance . . .*

Invitation

with thanks to Bob Cording

Where she lies on a gurney in Emergency
I read her a poem about lifting a small
plastic Spiderman from a ditch,

raising its arms to the sky as if calling
down a blessing. Suddenly her shut eyes
snap open,

and from the dark cave of her mouth
a strangely joyful noise.
She stares at cloud-white ceiling tiles.

Lament

- When I get to Emergency, they're piercing her for IV ports. Her hands are bleeding. Her mouth is open as if to scream *No no!* She whispers, "Just let me go."

- The ER room is S-21 – Sarah at 21 when we married 62 years ago. Or our address at 21 Goodrich Road in Simsbury before her Alzheimer's, a way station on the road to a farther home. However it is, this must be where she is meant to be.

- Her blood pressure stays direly low, despite IV fluids. Her body is in retreat from days of self-starvation in Memory Care.

- She rises to the sixth floor, has a view of stars and moon. In the morning the shadows of fumes from a smokestack, suntruck, dance on the building across from her, ascending.

- A nurse checking vitals shakes her head, explains in too much detail what is transpiring as if Sarah is an object, deaf. Though she barely speaks now, she says softly "bla ba-bla ba-bla-bla-bla" and adds "Too late, too late."

- The doctor says we must "let nature take its course." Sarah overhears him. A wide smile plays across her face.

- I am not myself. Being pushed in a wheelchair to my car by a staffer named Michael, I find myself singing "Michael, row the boat ashore, hallelujah . . ." It's a form of relief. Do I know the song refers to the Archangel Michael, who ferries souls of the dead to Heaven? I do know that something profound is at the heart of those lyrics. This ending we are part of deepens us.

• Sarah puckers her lips and opens her eyes to Granddaughter Emily and Grandson Mack, looks clear into the heart of each, whispers their names, and says, "I am so sorry."

• She calls Eleanor and Robin "my little babies," her voice distant, almost inaudible. Her azure eyes flicker. There are no words for her smile. *Beatific* is not sufficient.

• I show my darling a book I wrote for her, out just today. She looks at the photo of us on the back cover, taken two years ago. She absorbs it slowly through clouded eyes, then utters a soft cry of joy.

• Robin and Eleanot take turns lying next to their mother, closed parentheses. They nuzzle her cheek and neck as if to suckle. Their hands twine with hers.

• While Sarah seems to be napping, Robin reads aloud a poem containing the line "All is a blur." Suddenly she whispers "All is a blur," eyes searching.

• Sah calls from Colorado and speaks to her Mumsie, telling stories from the past in which her mother played such a central role, one of the stories being about a time when Sah and her sister were jealous of new-born Robin and were pacified when Sarah gave them nippled baby bottles filled with chocolate milk.

• On the sixth night of Sarah's preparation for her journey, a "Green Comet" streaks across the sky above St. Francis.

• Her lips tremble in time to chorales of Giovanni Palestrina broadcast on Robin's cell. She might be singing at St. Paul's in 1954. Her eyes flicker. I imagine she sees saints in a frieze or perhaps in person, part of a different choir she is already joining.

• Eleanor holds a tea bag of Lapsang Souchong to her Marm's nose, as I did when my own mother was dying. Sarah breathes it in, pulls it closer.

• Just hours from her departure, she continues to rest more serenely than she has for months. A rag doll elf from her friend Lorrie rests by her temple, and a Palm Sunday cross lies on the gold and russet prayer shawl covering her.

• Late on the seventh day, Robin and I drive home for a brief respite, leaving Eleanor to sit vigil. We eat a quick dinner next to an amaryllis blooming strangely for a second time, lit by my mother's lamp, which only a few people can work, Sarah being one of them. Suddenly the light flickers, then flickers again. "It is time," Robin says and rushes to St. Francis – as once, sitting by that light, I rose and rushed to the side of my father, just in time. Tonight I am grounded by my debility, as my mother was then. Thank God for Robin.

• Back beside Sarah, her breathing quickened and irregular, Robin joins Eleanor in reciting the Lord's Prayer and the 23rd Psalm for the second time that day, and now adds the words of "Now I Lay Me Down." After "I pray the Lord my soul to take" and Eleanor's telling her Marm that she will take care of husband Rennie, Sarah is free to leave and slips away so quietly and peacefully that it is at first unclear she is gone.

In Memoriam

for Sarah Couch McQuilkin (1938–2023)

• We are numb. All's a blur, as Sarah said, and work is perhaps
a saving grace. Robin and Eleanor clear her room at The
Meadows, so much of her making its journey to one home while
she completes her journey to another. *Michael, row your boat
ashore, hallelujah . . .* There are tears for the things returning:
her precious stuffed animals, the blinking Christmas tree, all
those gorgeous paintings . . .

• Sarah's children and I spend two days sobbing intermittently.
It takes very little to set us off: her wrist watch, whose hands
point to Saving Time, no longer possible; her coloring book
lighthouse with its beacon carefully filled in; her sparkling blue
cane the color of her eyes – I hold it to touch her hand.

• Then I am alone. Eleanor barely makes it home through a
fearful snow and wind storm, fit analogue for anguish, the same
storm that sends the smoke of Sarah's cremation far afield. I
breathe her in.

• I have sloughed off much of what once seemed important.
Nothing matters but finding ways of being with my Sarah. I
answer a myriad messages of condolence (so much love for her),
but in that continuing blur.

• I wear a life-saving pendant whose acronym is SARA . . .

• The children call to check on me. Eleanor wants to be sure I
am hydrating. I must do it for the children. So much love from
them. Robin says he has seen a solitary Hooded Merganser, a
white-headed male swimming by himself. Perhaps next time

there will be a courting pair of Mergansers, a swan-necked, cinnamon-tufted beauty joining the solitary male.

- I have my Sarah back. She sits in her earth-colored urn at the table where she always sat by me, looking out at the koi pond and its gardens.

- Her heart was so big I could perhaps squeeze my smaller heart into hers, be with her always.

The Lettering

Dust to the dust of earth, to particles of the air,
to currents of the river and lake, she will go
forth, join the elements, spell who she is and,
for a time, was.

Her ashes will be creaturely,
circling in the sky, landing in furrows of earth,
floating on the Farmington: shape of the beaver
she loved to see leaping in Pickerel Cove,

shape of the red fox
who left his prints in her garden, shape
of the golden finches, familiar souls she named:

animal shapes like hieroglyphs that change to
letters of an alphabet with which to say her good-
byes and hellos. Godspeed, Godspeed.

III. AFTERWORLD

Cold Morning

I take it as a sign, what I see on the pond:
a white drain pipe brought low as Lucifer,
reflected on the pond, limber above still-
stunned fish. It ripples on moving water

like a huge snake weaving toward stones
rimming the pond – the Serpent of Grief
retreating, I hope. Dear God, let it remain
in its dark den among the stones, relent.

Let the world turn, my grieving cease.
May the only truth be white snowdrops,
crocus gold, first chancing of a daffodil.
But the Serpent of Grief persists . . .

More deeply, I know it is salvation.
The bite of grief creates the knot
that ties me to my belovèd, the sure sign
we will never separate. I welcome grief in.

Afterlife

Hunched over on my too-small scooter
like the curled and grizzled Tollund Man
preserved by properties of his burial bog,
his noose-necked body looking almost
alive, I make my rounds, trying to stay
connected to the old ways with Sarah.

I reset the tall, untimely clock, wind its lead
weights higher as I did while she waited
patiently, keeping me from dropping the key
to the unreachable base of the time machine;
and water – without her to prune – the peace
lily with its white spathes reaching to heaven.

I lose time more and more, unkempt and
cramped. I'm tempted by transit
to Sarah's timeless, choreless, choral world.

Migration

Listening to *Scheherazade*, the Shipwreck movement,
on this sixth-week anniversary of my dear one's death,
I founder, hit bottom, see so much treasure lost.
Good God! I push off, rise to the surface,

and look to riches remaining: an earth-brown urn
with a numbered medallion on top – dog tag certifying
she fought her war, has earned her rest;
the copy of *Wind in the Willows* I read by her bedside;

and a wild goose, base of a lamp by which my mother
lit her way to the underworld.
Around the neck of the goose on a hospital band
hang two rings from the stilled hand of my Belovèd,

doubly a blessing
in light of the grief we felt at losing our first wedding
rings, eased off past swollen knuckles and stashed
somewhere forgotten.

In the enchantment of *Scheherazade*, I look to
the Canada Goose bearing new rings, poised for flight
I could join. It is migration time, season for reunion.

Pancake Heaven

How could I, mourning,
be such a glutton
for cakes today
in Pancake Heaven?

If only I had you by me,
my love, I'd be in heaven.
As it is, I am merely
allaying my aloneness,

staving off the removal
of staves holding the Spirit
in my cask of a body.

In lieu of that I send this –
the purest love instilled
in my grief

like the "angel's share"
evaporating from a cask
of aging single malt.

Sea Thistle

I have pulled the last gold from your
memorial arrangement, my dearest –
a yellow rose crinkled as the corsage
you kept in water long after our first
dance. In this latter day bouquet,

only the blues remain, but look –
the up-reaching lapis lazuli arms of
the enduring sea thistles point to
a new sort of mourning, their startling
blues akin to the resilience I feel,

admiring the artistry of our fine grave
stone, our names lying one over the other,
in lieu of my second date, a space. Just
now, my dear, I will try to fill it in with
more than a number – for those we love.

The Homing

A soft night-breeze winds about the apart-
ment, calling to mind the sound
of wind in willows, then the book itself . . .

I read to my love from *Wind in the Willows*
at Christmas, a month before her passing
to the home she had yearned for so long –

the chapter entitled "Dulce Domum"
(sweet home) in which Mole, having been
up from underground all summer, carousing,

wants his old burrow, for which he longs
so fiercely he sobs when he smells it nearby.
I will always hear her own sob of joy

when Mole enters "Mole End." I hope she
sensed from the break in my voice
how well I understood the depth of her need.

Taking Her In

I treasure whatever Sarah wore most recently,
and closest to herself – slippers, socks, undershirts,
pajamas, beanies – the more unwashed the better.
I bury my face in the scent of her, wear whatever
of hers I can. I throw her prayer shawl over my head,
wrap her ams around me. I take her in.

Screensaver

Good morning, my love. Wish you were here
to dispel the weather: a gale, freezing rain, 38°.
Alexa promises I can "expect more of the same."
PBS adds "tornadic activity" in Mississippi has
killed 29, and many are gone from the explosion
of a chocolate factory in Pennsylvania.
Expecting more of the same, I am thinking
back to a brief glimpse of ruby sun through half-
open blinds at 6 a.m., then Schumann's
Scenes from Childhood. And now this photograph
on my screensaver – you at one in your stroller:
sun-round face and widely welcoming smile.
Please, more of the same.

The Rift

Searching for a few joyful
memories of her
in the place optimistically
known as The Meadows,

I get as far as Reception –
where I collapse. I cannot . . .
cannot visit her old haunts.
She is not there, not anywhere!

In today's breaking news
a jagged fissure has ripped
acres of olive trees
into a rock-ridden chasm.

It will be years before anything
can grow in that rift or the rift
in my heart, broken open.

A reporter speaks of nature's
healing power. I want to believe.

Transport

Just three months ago we went on your first
outing since being immured in Memory Care.
The entry to Podiatry was dark, elevator kaput,

and we resorted to stairs like Everest climbers,
clumping, gripping the railing, but arrived
at a sort of heavenly office, brightly lit...

There, prone without you today, looking down
on my bent and corned club toes
and grayly elephantine feet, I close my eyes,

am transported to you beside me back then,
being trimmed, your long, elegant feet
in the pink. After the clipping,

I suggested that we go out for tea and pastries.
The elevator worked and we found our way
to a Millennials' café... Today,

I almost fall getting to the car. But I reach
our café, engage in one-way remembering,
am transported to Portugal, just wed,

savoring espresso and *pastel de nata* together,
not believing our good fortune
and you creating a sensation wherever we go.

Ash Wednesday

Please! I hear from the brown
plastic urn they've put you in

who hated confinement.
I cut the seal, indecent

as Good Housekeeping's stamp . . .
Oh, how finely white your ash!

You can breathe now.

It being Ash Wednesday, I fix
you to my forehead to say

I wish I'd done better by you.

I furrow my brow. On it, this
baptism by a puckering
of finger-wetted ash, a kissing.

On Not Dying Just Yet

I lay me down after a day
of longing for Sarah,
a part of me asking the Lord
my soul to take.

At dawn, not taken,
like Queequeg in *Moby Dick* –
who lies down in his canoe-coffin
but recalls something he must do,

lifts the paddle and harpoon
next to him, steps from the coffin,
and goes on – I too
lower feet to the floor, wobble up

with cane and Sharpie in hand, and
over coffee try to strike right words
for a memo to her in the new world.

The Sweetening

If anyone heard me talking to you, my love,
(nowhere to be seen except in the apartment
of my heart) in that Bloomfield parking lot,
I trust they assumed I had a Bluetooth.

Actually, as I walked to the little bakery
we used to visit, it was a *sweet* tooth I had
and your even sweeter tooth in mind.
"Today," I said, "let's have blueberry muffins."

Speaking of sweets, dear Sarah –
during our pastor's visit yesterday, when I said
I'd been less than an ideal spouse, I heard

your sweet *We all* . . . in his. Looking up,
I saw what I hadn't before, God knows why –
on our moribund orchid a purple triptych of
fragrant petals with more to come.

Potter's Wheel, First Day of Spring

Good morning, my dearest. You're still
with me today – nine spoonfuls' worth
of ash in the clay turkey pot you built.
Our son cradled the rest gently, carried it

to the river bend where fifty years ago
you spread a checkered tablecloth at noon
and we saw how far we could skip stones.
There, he and your kin scattered palmfuls

over the water, your white ash sailing out
like winnowed wheat or a spreading net,
drifting down and circling in the current
on your way to the Sea. Still, bits of bone

glitter like mica in wet clay by the river's eddy,
perfect medium. I see you once more working
the clay, fading into God at His potter's wheel.
What to make of you? A dove, an owl, a breeze . . .

Wind in the Chimney

(Easter, 2023)

His chimney pots sing in a swirl of breeze
like your swirl in the river where he freed
your ash, my belovèd,
and saw its lightest chaff curl into the sky.

Our son wonders at the chiming
from his chimney, then slowly knows: the tone
is a whetted fingertip's circling a wineglass rim,
rising from a low hum to the highest pitch

you performed to celebrate family gatherings.
He blesses an urge toward words in this music
of wind against the rims of his pots: a slurred,
incipient "I love you," words you whispered

when you ended, all of us by the bed inheriting
words never to be lost, circling above us forever.

Snowy Owl

I look up, see you at home on the risers
of your new choir,
top row, taller than the others, a nimbus
of startling white hair framing high-boned
Nordic features and azure eyes,
voice a part of the whole yet purely itself.

I am reminded of Snowy Owls
you and I encountered – in Mont-Dore
on the Massif, and later on the wild shore
of Lake Ontario. The first, mid-road, stood

her ground; the second gradually rose
on deliberate legs, another hunting ground
in mind, and flew in a white blur. So it is with
you, my belovèd, risen to your own far world
but near, near, always in the haven of my heart.

ABOUT THE AUTHOR

Rennie McQuilkin was Poet Laureate of Connecticut from 2015 to 2018. His work has appeared in *The Atlantic, Poetry, The Southern Review, The Yale Review, The Hudson Review, The American Scholar,* and elsewhere. This is his twenty-first poetry collection. He has received a number of awards for his work, including a fellowship from the National Endowment for the Arts and six fellowships from the Connecticut Commission on the Arts, as well as a Lifetime Achievement Award from the Connecticut Center for the Book. In 2010 his volume of new and selected poems, *The Weathering,* was awarded the Center's annual poetry prize under the aegis of the Library of Congress; and in 2018, *North of Eden* received the Next Generation Indie Book Award in Poetry. For nine years he directed the Sunken Garden Poetry Festival, which he co-founded at Hill-Stead Museum in Farmington, CT. In 2018, he and his wife of sixty-two years – artist, teacher, counselor, and gardener Sarah McQuilkin – moved to the Seabury retirement community in Bloomfield, CT. They are the parents of three wonderful children. Unhappily, Sarah passed away in January, 2023.

This book is set in Garamond Premier Pro, which had its genesis in 1988 when type-designer Robert Slimbach visited the Plantin-Moretus Museum in Antwerp, Belgium, to study its collection of Claude Garamond's metal punches and typefaces. During the fifteen hundreds, Garamond – a Parisian punch-cutter – produced a refined array of book types that combined an unprecedented degree of balance and elegance, for centuries standing as the pinnacle of beauty and practicality in type-founding. They were based on the handwriting of Angelo Vergecio, court librarian of the French king Francis I. Slimbach has created a new interpretation based on Garamond's designs and on compatible italics cut by Robert Granjon, Garamond's contemporary.

This book is available at Amazon and other bookstores
and inscribed copies can be ordered
from Rennie McQuilkin
400 Seabury Dr., Apt. 5196
Bloomfield, CT 06002.
Send $16 per book
plus $4 shipping
by check payable
to the author.

•

For more information on the work of Rennie McQuilkin
visit www.antrimhousebooks.com/authors.html.
The author can be contacted at
RMcQuil36@gmail.com
and 860.519.1804.

CPSIA information can be obtained
at www.ICGtesting.com
Printed in the USA
LVHW100032120423
744085LV00013B/45

9 798986 552279